FROM
INTROSPECTION
TO ACTION

Enjoy the
journey.
Dr Nicole

FROM INTROSPECTION TO ACTION

The High Level Professional's
28 Day Journey to Improving Mental Health

Nicole B. Washington, DO, MPH

FROM INTROSPECTION TO ACTION
Published by Purposely Created Publishing Group™
Copyright © 2018 Nicole Washington

All rights reserved.

Printed in the United States of America
ISBN: 978-1-948400-30-5

Special discounts are available on bulk quantity purchases by book clubs, associations and special interest groups. For details email: sales@publishyourgift.com or call (888) 949-6228.

For information logon to:
www.PublishYourGift.com

"The only person who can pull me down is myself, and I'm not going to let myself pull me down anymore"

—C. Joybell C.

DEDICATION

This book is dedicated to all you busy business professionals out there who need to take a step back and engage in some self-care. You work day in and day out, often leaving very little time for you. You know who you are!

You can't remember the last time you did something just for yourself. You have hobbies and interests you used to love that you vow to pick back up when you have the time. You have hobbies you would like to take up but are still waiting on. So, do you know when that will be? Never! Why? Because you can't sit still. You don't feel comfortable unless you are busy and active and involved in something. You may not even be able to separate your identity from your career anymore. Yes, you are a doctor, lawyer, or C-Suite executive, but there is also a person in there, beyond the title. A person who needs just as much attention as your family or career does.

Let's face it: your careers are demanding and, if you have a family on top, things can feel downright overwhelming. Sometimes you feel like you can't have one more thing put on your plate or you might snap, so you put yourself on the back burner. Maybe you have an untreated mental health disorder. Maybe you are just in a funk and need to take some time to evaluate your mental health and make minor changes.

Whatever the case, this book is for you! I pray that its chapters give you the opportunity to take some time out for you. Give yourself a little mental health checkup, learn new concepts, refresh your knowledge, and spend the next 28 days investing in one of your most valuable assets: your mental health. You'll be glad you did!

TABLE OF CONTENTS

PREFACE

This book was born from a place of extreme uneasiness in my life. I was married to the man of my dreams, had two beautiful kids, and was a working a psychiatrist, a career that I had been working towards since I was a kid. Yet, I was extremely unhappy and couldn't figure out why. I was stressed, overwhelmed, and spending so much time working on and for everyone else that I totally forgot about myself. I was irritable, not sleeping well, and completely in denial about how fragile I was. I was holding on by a thread and couldn't see it. That's right! I am a psychiatrist and couldn't see that I needed an intervention. I've always had a million things going on at once and multitasked myself into the ground. But I was still functioning, so I kept pushing through.

Then, when I was at a visit with my primary care physician, she said to me, "Girl, you are doing so much. Are you okay? Are you taking care of yourself?" At that moment, I paused and cried like a child who just had her favorite toy taken away. I left that appointment with a whole new view of myself. I was not quite as great as I thought I was! I also realized that I had two choices: to either stay in a grinding rut or to make changes to improve my quality of life.

I soon started paying attention to other professionals who I came in contact with and quickly saw that I was not alone. Several of my acquaintances and friends, all business professionals, were struggling with similar feelings and problems. We are all overachieving, multitasking monsters who tend to spend little time on ourselves. Some of them are actively involved in psychiatric treatment, some of them aren't but should be, and some of them just need to take a little time out to do some self-reflection. This book was created for all of us!

INTRODUCTION

This book will take you on a four-week journey that will include a little bit of education, a whole lot of introspection, and the empowerment to take action. While this book was designed for the high-achieving professional, its topics are beneficial to many. Every reading will not apply to you personally, but you can gain something from each. It might also give you some perspective into the behaviors of others around you.

You will spend ten to fifteen minutes per day, reading about a different topic and reflecting on what you have read, asking yourself these questions below:

- Does this reading apply to me?

- Does this reading apply to someone I know?

⊙ Can I take anything from this reading and apply it to my life? If so, how?

You may have some additional reflection questions associated with each day's reading.

Week 1 focuses on general mental health concepts. You will learn about "normal" moods, the differences between depression and bipolar disorders, the importance of sleep, addictions, social media and its effects on your mental health, and personality disorders.

Week 2 and 3 cover destructive, unhealthy thoughts that can have negative effects on your mood and anxiety. We will go through some of the most common negative thoughts that people experience and learn ways to deal with them more appropriately.

Week 4 is action time! You will learn about the importance of self-care, boundary setting, acceptance of your broken self, gratitude, and options for mental health care. At the end of this week, you will create your mental health plan using information that we've covered up until then

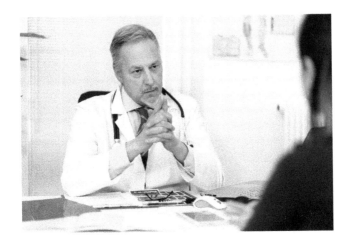

So, You Want to Be a Psychiatrist

By the end of this week, you won't exactly have attained the knowledge gained by a psychiatry residency, but you will have learned basic mental health concepts and be able to reasonably discuss the most common disorders.

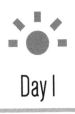

Day 1

WHAT IS A NORMAL MOOD?

What is your definition of a "normal" mood? Take some time think about your answer. If you define a normal mood based on happiness, you might find yourself with an unrealistic view of what a normal mood really is. Happiness is great, but imagine if we were happy all of the time despite what is happening in our lives. That would make for some unusual situations.

A normal mood actually consists of a wide range of emotions including anger, sadness, and fear, just to name a few. It is perfectly appropriate to experience anger if someone cuts you off in traffic or sadness if you experience a loss. The problem presents when the expression of these emotions is either above and beyond what is typically expected or if the resulting emotion lasts longer than you'd expect. For instance, if someone upsets you during a meeting at work and you break a vase in your office, that is over-expression above and beyond what is typically expected and an indication of a disorder.

For most of us, happiness is pleasant, so we don't mind experiencing it. The same cannot be said for other emotions. It can be very uncomfortable to feel sadness, anger, or fear. This is especially difficult for many high-achieving professionals because these feelings tend to come with a sense of a loss of control, which is tough for people who tend to thrive on maintaining control of most situations. We may even choose to use defense mechanisms like humor to avoid dealing with the uncomfortable emotion. However, it's important to allow yourself to feel uncomfortable feelings so that you can learn how to navigate them appropriately.

POINTS TO PONDER:

🡢 What is your definition of a normal mood?

🡢 Which emotions cause you the most discomfort?

🡢 What tactics (humor, changing subject, avoidance) do you find yourself using to avoid dealing with uncomfortable emotions?

NOTES

NOTES

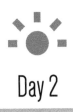

Day 2

MOOD DISORDERS

When we think of mood disorders, we typically refer to major depressive disorder or bipolar disorder. Major depressive disorder consists of a depressive episode that lasts at least two weeks and can be characterized by changes in sleep pattern, loss of interests in previously enjoyed activities, low energy, impaired memory/concentration, appetite changes, feelings of extreme guilt, feelings of worthlessness, hopelessness, and suicidal thoughts. A person doesn't have to experience all of these to receive a diagnosis of depression. The level of impairment will determine the level of severity of the disorder, which can be treated with medication, psychotherapy, or a combination of both.

Bipolar disorder is characterized by depressive episodes described above, as well as either manic or hypomanic episodes. It is much more than just having mood swings. These episodes of mania or hypomania last for several days and include distinct periods of time with either persistently elevated, irritable, or expansive moods and increased energy. Other symptoms include pressured speech or talkativeness, racing thoughts, increased self-esteem or grandiosity, decreased need for sleep to feel rested, being easily distracted, and increased engagement in goal-directed activities or activities that may bring pleasure but have high potential for negative consequences (i.e. promiscuity or shopping sprees).

These manic episodes would be very different than the person's usual mood, which is important to note because someone who has a more pervasive problem with promiscuity or excessive spending is likely not experiencing manic episodes. There is also another form of bipolar disorder with similar episodes that don't last as long or cause as much impairment. The typical recommendation for treatment of bipolar disorder is mood stabilizing medication.

POINTS TO PONDER:

Review the following checklists to see if you might be suffering from a mood disorder:

_____ Depression Checklist (Episode of at least two weeks):

_____ Depressed mood most of the day (either described by self or noticed by others).

_____ Decreased interest in activities you used to enjoy.

_____ Sleep disturbance (either increase or decrease).

_____ Appetite changes (either increase or decrease) or unexplained weight changes.

_____ Fatigue or loss of energy.

_____ Feelings of worthlessness or excessive, inappropriate guilt.

_____ Impaired memory or concentration.

_____ Recurrent thoughts of death or suicidal thoughts.

If you checked five or more of these, consider engaging in treatment. If you are experiencing feelings of worthlessness or suicidal thoughts, absolutely engage in treatment, regardless of whether the other symptoms apply or not.

MANIA CHECKLIST (EPISODE OF MULTIPLE DAYS):

_____ Increased self-esteem or grandiose thoughts.

_____ Decreased need for sleep (feeling rested after only a couple of hours).

_____ Talking more than usual or faster than usual.

_____ Racing thoughts.

_____ Easily distracted.

_____ Increase in goal-directed activities.

_____ Involvement in activities without regard to consequences (sex, spending, gambling, etc.).

If you have experienced at least three of these during a distinct period of time, along with elevated, expansive, or irritable mood, you may be experiencing symptoms of bipolar disorder.

NOTES

NOTES

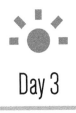

Day 3

PERSONALITY DISORDERS

Some illnesses are episodic and others are more pervasive, like personality disorders. Personality disorder symptoms are more chronic, indicate a pattern of behavior that strays from the population norm, and cause distress or impairment. A few of the more prevalent personality disorders are borderline personality disorder, narcissistic personality disorder, and obsessive compulsive personality disorder.

Borderline personality disorder is known for patterns of instability related to interpersonal relationships and self-image. Individuals with this disorder tend to have an unstable sense of who they are, which lead to seemingly sudden changes in goals, values, or career. They may be impulsive and have recurrent suicidal or self-harm behavior such as cutting, intense mood swings, anger outbursts, and chronic feelings of emptiness. People with borderline personality disorder may be misdiagnosed as bipolar disorder due to the similarities between symptoms. Remember that bipolar disorder is an episodic illness, whereas personality disorders are more constant.

Narcissistic personality disorder is characterized by a need for admiration, lack of empathy, and grandiosity. These individuals may have an inflated sense of importance and entitlement, exhibit arrogance, and require a high level of admiration. They tend to believe that they are special and that they should mostly, if not exclusively, associate with other special people of high status. Relationships suffer for those with narcissistic personality disorder due to their arrogance, need for admiration, and habit of taking advantage of others for their own gain.

Obsessive compulsive personality disorder (OCPD) is one of the most prevalent personality disorders and one that overlaps with type-A personality characteristics, making it the one that will resonate most with high-level professionals. Those with OCPD have a tendency to maintain control through preoccupation with details, rules, lists, schedules, and order, so much so that the level of perfectionism makes it difficult to actually complete the task at hand. I see this in physicians who have difficulty completing medical records in a timely manner. They usually have such strict standards of how the notes should be completed that it takes an unusually long period of time for them to complete said notes. Those with OCPD may also put off engaging in personal time because they are too busy or they may take work with them on vacation so no time is wasted. Those with OCPD are also hesitant to delegate task to others due to their concern that things will not be completed exactly the way they want them. The great majority of us will see some of these characteristics in ourselves.

POINTS TO PONDER:

⊙ Do you find it difficult to let others help you when engaging in a project or task?

⊙ Do you have a difficult time leaving work at work?

⊙ Do you identify with any of the characteristics above? If yes, which ones?

TIPS FOR DEALING WITH OCPD SYMPTOMS:

⊙ Focus on the enjoyable parts of activities, not the rules.

⊙ Avoid the temptation to bring work life into true leisure time on a regular basis.

⊙ Engage in an activity that you aren't good at but think you might enjoy.

⊙ Set parameters on your phone so that email notifications don't keep coming in through the evening.

NOTES

NOTES

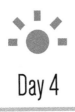

Day 4

FUNCTIONAL ADDICTIONS

When we think of people with addictions, we tend to think of those who use drugs or alcohol excessively with obvious impairment related to their use. We don't think of high-level professionals with functional addictions, or addictions that don't seem to be all that impairing on the surface. Such people can have significant substance use problems without them being overt. Those who are high-functioning can spend several years hiding their substance use or finding ways to justify their use because of the demanding nature of their work. If they can additionally continue to fulfill work and family obligations, their addiction can go unnoticed or will be thought of as "okay" because of the lack of obvious impairment.

Getting treatment for an addiction can be a scary thing to pursue, one that requires a level of self-honesty that typically isn't there. After all, denial is huge with those who are dealing with functional addictions. Stigma is another barrier to seeking treatment: we worry about what others will say or think about us. If you are in a public position, there is the concern of losing your status in the community or even your job as a result of being honest about your addiction. While these concerns are all reasonable, the largest concern should be the potential negative health consequences of long-term alcohol or drug use, such as liver disease or cognitive impairment.

Treatment of substance use disorders can be on an inpatient or outpatient basis. Outpatient treatment can encompass everything from twelve-step meetings to traditional individual outpatient treatment to intensive programs that provide group treatment multiple times per week for a defined period of time. For those who have failed outpatient treatment or those who have a more severe addiction, inpatient treatment may be necessary. Keep in mind that inpatient treatment requires more of a commitment (though well worth it) since it requires you to be away from job and family for an extended period of time.

POINTS TO PONDER:

Could you be suffering with addiction?

_____ Do you use illicit drugs or prescription drugs that are not prescribed to you?

_____ Are you a woman who drinks more than one drink per day?

_____ Are you a man who drinks more than two drinks per day?

_____ Do you find that you require alcohol or drugs to relax?

_____ Do you use drinking as a reward for a rough day?

_____ Have you ever had periods of blackout while drinking?

_____ Do you drink more than you intend to?

_____ Have you had to call in to work or been late due to a night of heavy drinking or drug use?

_____ If you miss a day or two of drinking, do you experience shakes, sweats, nausea, or increased anxiety?

_____ Have you had to drink more to achieve the same level of intoxication or have you noticed that you don't get as intoxicated as you used to, despite consuming the same amount?

If you checked any of these items, you should consider seeking an expert opinion on whether or not you meet criteria for a substance use disorder.

NOTES

NOTES

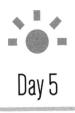

Day 5

SLEEP MATTERS

A good night of sleep is so important! Let me repeat that for those of you who live by the "I'll sleep when I'm dead" creed: a good night of sleep is so important. Achieving adequate rest allows you to restore and refresh for a new day. When you don't get the sleep that your body needs, it can lead to impaired concentration and increase in mistakes on the job. For some lines of work, these mistakes can be a matter of life or death. Did you know that driving on little sleep can be just as impairing, if not more, as driving intoxicated? Lack of sleep can also have negative consequences to your physical health, such as increases in cardiovascular problems, weight gain, and immune system impairment.

Sometimes, this sleep interruption is due to you pushing yourself to get more work done or playing catch up. Other times, this is due to symptoms of depression, anxiety, or substance use. And still other times, it's just a reflection of having a stressful day. Whatever the reason, you can take simple steps to enhance your quality of sleep.

Ways to improve your sleep hygiene:

- Avoid spending extended periods of time in bed other than for sleep or sex.

- Engage in aerobic exercise during the day to improve sleep at night.

- Cut off caffeine and nicotine in the evening to avoid sleep disruption.

- Avoid lengthy naps. But remember that a short power nap can help improve performance.

- Avoid foods that cause heartburn close to bed time.

- Take hot baths to help induce sleepiness.

⊙ Avoid alcohol close to bedtime.

⊙ If you can't fall asleep after twenty minutes, get up and do something relaxing until you feel sleepy again, then try going back to sleep.

POINTS TO PONDER:

⊙ Most adults require seven to eight hours of sleep per night. Do you get this amount on a consistent basis?

⊙ Do you wake up feeling rested?

⊙ Are you able to stay awake throughout the day without dozing off?

If you answered "no" to any of these questions, you may not be achieving adequate sleep and may benefit from reviewing the sleep hygiene list above to see what changes you can make to have positive effects on your sleep pattern. If these don't work, you may want to follow up with your primary care physician and request a sleep study.

NOTES

NOTES

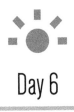

Day 6

SOCIAL MEDIA AND MENTAL HEALTH

Social media has allowed us to connect with people in ways we never have before. It can be a great way to keep in touch with family and friends we don't see often and to reconnect with those we've lost touch with along the way. However, too much social media can have negative effects on our mental health.

First, we can develop addictions to the internet. This is a new concept that's still being extensively researched but it's thought to be similar to drug and alcohol addictions. You may feel a certain rush of endorphins when you hear that notification alert and have a hard time resisting the urge to check your phone or computer. You may also spend more time scrolling through your news feed than you anticipated, which can be distracting and cause you to be unproductive at work. This decrease in productivity can put undue stress on an already stressful day leading to anxiety and/or low mood.

Social media can also create a bad case of FOMO, or Fear of Missing Out. FOMO occurs when you see someone's social media post and you start to play the comparison game. You question your own life based upon what you've seen. You may see a colleague post something and become focused on comparing their work life to yours or the size of their house to yours. You might also sign up for activities that really don't fit into your schedule, just because you try to seize every opportunity your peers are engaging in. Given these symptoms, FOMO can lead to anxiety, low mood, low self-esteem, and increased stress load trying to keep up.

POINTS TO PONDER:

- ❯ Do you check your social media accounts throughout the day while at work?

- ❯ When you hear a notification on your phone, do you find it necessary to check it right away?

I challenge you to a social media fast, just to determine if you spend an excessive amount of time on social media sites throughout the day. For the next work day, no social media checking. No posting, no scrolling the newsfeed. If you find that you must stop yourself from grabbing your phone multiple times per day, then you could benefit from modifying your social media intake using the tips below:

- ❯ Set defined times throughout the day, during which you allow yourself to browse social media.

- ❯ Turn off notification alerts from social media accounts to decrease the urge to check.

- ❯ No posting during the work day to avoid the urge to check for comments, likes, etc.

NOTES

NOTES

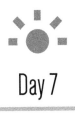

Day 7

TREATMENT OPTIONS

There are several treatment options for your mental health. You can do nothing (which really isn't a good option), manage medication, receive psychotherapy, or pursue a combination of both medication and therapy.

Despite the fact that doing nothing is detrimental to your mental health, people often choose to not seek services. For high-level professionals, the barriers to seeking treatment typically include lack of time, stigma, and concerns about medication interfering with functioning. In more demanding career fields, it is difficult to find time during regular hours to seek treatment, especially when most treatment offices are only open during regular hours. Furthermore, no matter how much we try to educate communities about mental illness, stigma remains a huge hindrance. If you are a recognizable face in your community, you may be hesitant to be seen going into a psychiatrist or therapist's office. However, please be aware that the negative consequences of untreated mental health disorders outweigh appearances. Not only will you possibly have decreased productivity due to functional impairment but you could also experience an increased risk in substance use disorders, heart disease, weight gain, and relationship dysfunction.

Medication can be used to treat most psychiatric disorders. There are multiple classes of drugs that are used to treat mood disorders, anxiety, and psychosis, and it is also not uncommon for a psychiatrist to use a drug in a way that is not necessarily indicated by the FDA. This is a common standard of care: after a drug's release, it can be discovered that it's components are beneficial for uses outside of its original purpose, and doctors successfully use it to treat other conditions.

Typically, when starting a new medication, you will be asked to come in for a follow-up two to four weeks later and then visits every four weeks thereafter. Once you start to see significant improvements, your visits may be spread out to every three months, or even every six months in some cases. This is at the discretion of your outpatient psychiatrist. It is important that you have conversations up front about medications and their side effects so that you can make an informed decision about taking certain drugs or not. Make it very clear to the physician that you want to avoid medication that can be sedating, in order to avoid further functional impairment.

Psychotherapy, or talk therapy, can occur individually or in group settings, depending upon the nature of the treatment. In general, psychotherapy helps you identify any dysfunctional thoughts, behaviors, or emotions, and then guides you through changing them in order to improve functioning.

You may seek out therapy if you have a major disorder such as depression, bipolar disorder, anxiety, or a substance use disorder. In addition, you may also seek out therapy to help get through a rough patch in your life, such as in job performance. If you're a physician who had a bad outcome or an attorney going through a difficult case, you might consider seeking out brief psychotherapy to help with the emotional distress of that period in your career.

The combination of psychotherapy and medication management has been shown to be superior to either treatment alone for several conditions.

POINTS TO PONDER:

- Have you previously considered talking to a therapist or seeking mental health treatment, but changed your mind? If so, what were the reasons?

- What personal struggles do you have that could be addressed through therapy?

- Have you ever considered medication treatment for mental health disorder?

NOTES

NOTES

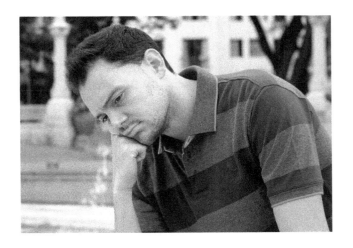

WEEK 2 AND 3

Tackling Dysfunctional Thoughts

Over the next two weeks, we will focus on common dysfunctional thoughts that can lead to low mood, anxiety, and overall functional impairment. Your thoughts have a lot of power in guiding your emotions, so understanding dysfunctional ones will help you reexamine how you think about yourself, how you relate to the world around you, and how those things affect your overall mental health.

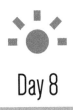

Day 8

HOLDING YOURSELF TO UNREASONABLY HIGH STANDARDS

Robert is an advertising executive who had a presentation to give to a potential client. When he got to one of his slides, his mind went blank and he stumbled over his words. Still, he was able to recover and complete the presentation without further hiccups. He ended up landing the account and the client thanked him for the hard work he put into the process. Nevertheless, Robert was very upset about the moment he stumbled over some words. He stated to a peer that he was certain that the VP of the company thought he was an idiot after the presentation. Later that night, Robert drank heavily to deal with his frustration.

Most people who are very successful don't just get there overnight. I am guessing that you are no different. You've likely held yourself to high standards since you were in grade school and this has carried over into your career. You may be guilty of convincing yourself that, when you make even a seemingly small mistake, others will think negatively of you and your ability to perform at a high level.

There is absolutely nothing wrong with setting the bar high; however, there is something wrong with not leaving yourself room to be human. You will make mistakes. You will miss the mark and will not always bring your A-game into the office. *Everyone* makes mistakes. But your mistakes do not define you as a professional nor do they define you as a person.

POINTS TO PONDER

⊙ Can you recall the last time you made a mistake in the workplace? What happened?

⊙ How did you react? What thoughts did you have about yourself during that time?

⊙ If your thoughts were negative, how could you change them to something more realistic and less negative?

NOTES

NOTES

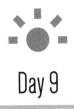

Day 9

FOCUSING ON THE NEGATIVE

Jan is a family medicine physician and her office is completing patient satisfaction surveys this week on random patients. Of the ten surveys that she received, nine of them were extremely positive with glowing comments. But one of them gave her low ratings and stated their unhappiness with her doctoring style. Jan could not stop thinking about this negative survey, despite the fact that 90% of the surveys were excellent. She spent all day talking about the feedback at work and continued to talk about it at home in the evening. When her husband asked her about the other surveys, she became upset, which lead to a huge argument.

When you focus on the negative, you tend to completely overlook all of the positive things that happened over the course of the day. This takes your thoughts to a very dark place where it becomes hard to see the positive things any longer, which can lead to irritability, interpersonal issues, low self-esteem, and increase in anxiety.

POINTS TO PONDER:

If you are guilty of concentrating on the negative, try this exercise:

Make a list of negative things that happened today and number them. For each of the negative things that happened today, write a positive thing that happened. Repeating this exercise during times that you find yourself dwelling on the negative can help keep your thoughts and goals straight, and hopefully prevent dysfunctional behaviors.

NOTES

NOTES

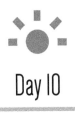

Day 10

I FEEL,
THEREFORE I AM

Jerry is a private banker and is one of five bankers in his department. In a meeting recently, a topic came up that Jerry had no prior knowledge of; however, all of his peers appeared to know what was going on. Jerry started to feel very anxious, like he was inferior to his coworkers. He continued to dwell on his inferiority and worried that this might lead him to lose his job. As a result, he worked late hours and took on more work in efforts to prove that he can handle the job.

Your feelings don't always reflect reality. Just because you feel inferior, doesn't mean that you are.

The danger of allowing your emotions to define reality is that you find yourself creating false realities that lead to anxiety or the worsening of existing anxiety symptoms. It can also lead to significant interpersonal issues, especially if a negative emotion leads you to believe inaccuracies about other people.

The best way to deal with situations like these is to change what you tell yourself. In the case of Jerry: instead of telling himself that he is inferior and in danger of losing his job, he could have told himself that he had somehow missed that information and now has the opportunity to learn about it and figure it out.

Even if you find yourself thinking the worst, remind yourself that those feelings are likely to pass. Being aware of that will be much more helpful than running nowhere with your thoughts.

POINTS TO PONDER:

→ Can you think of a time when your feelings on a topic were not representative of reality?

→ Do you find yourself experiencing anxious feelings in certain situation at work? If so, which ones? How do they affect your performance?

NOTES

NOTES

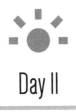

Day II

SHOULDA, WOULDA, COULDA

Since having her last child several years ago, Sherri has been struggling with her weight. She just recently started a diet and has trouble sticking with the plan. While at a kid's birthday party, she ate a cupcake and immediately felt bad about it. On the way home, she kept saying, "I shouldn't have eaten that cupcake." By the time she neared home, she was in tears and had to pull over to gather herself.

Making "should/shouldn't" statements indicate that things have to be the way that you expect them to be or else something is wrong. When you impose these nearly impossible rules on yourself and then go against them, you feel guilty, angry, and hard on yourself. These types of statements may also lead to interpersonal discord when you try to put the same rules onto other people, who will inevitably disappoint you because the rules only exist in your head.

"Have to" statements can also be thrown into this category. It is not uncommon for people to talk about what they "have to" do as if they are written in law, only to be extremely disappointed in themselves if that task or obligation doesn't get done.

POINTS TO PONDER

- What "should/shouldn't" rules do you have for yourself?

- What "should/shouldn't" rules do you tend to impose on other people?

- What are healthier ways to motivate yourself to do the things that you "should" do?

NOTES

NOTES

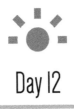

Day 12

HOLDING YOURSELF RESPONSIBLE

Darryl, a physician, received word that a patient died secondary to complications associated with diabetes. Darryl reviewed the chart multiple times that day, heavily critiquing himself on his treatment plan for the patient. He told his nurse, "Maybe if I had changed his meds at the last visit, this wouldn't have happened." This led to a high level of guilt and anxiety in Darryl's future patient interactions. He began constantly second-guessing himself in visits with patients and often looked up information in literature that he was very capable of treating from memory.

When you hold yourself responsible for events that aren't completely under your control, you will feel a significant amount of guilt and doubt yourself and your abilities. A great deal of high-achieving professionals like to have control over situations, but it is hard to have control over anyone other than yourself. Especially if you work with the public, this is a stressful relationship to deal with: if you are a physician like Darryl, you want to take care of your patients and help them get better, but you must also keep in mind that you can't be with that person around the clock or be personally responsible for decisions they may make.

POINTS TO PONDER:

Think of a personal relationship you have that is either strained or has ended due to conflict. Make a list of your wrongs and a list of the other person's wrongs in the situation. Repeat this same activity for a work-related incident. Identify, in both situations, what you can do to work on your errors and try to address one of the wrongs at your next opportunity.

Whether you are holding yourself completely responsible for something not under your control or you are absolving yourself from responsibility in a situation that you do have control over, the exercise above will address your issues. Take the time to see your side in the conflict and make the necessary moves to correct the situation if it's still possible.

NOTES

NOTES

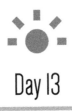

Day 13

DOWNPLAYING YOUR POSITIVES AND BLOWING UP YOUR MISTAKES

Jessica is a judge who recently received a humanitarian award for her work with disabled children. After the awards ceremony, she was complimented and congratulated for her work. However, she responded with statements like, "Well, I was assigned that docket so I was just doing my job" or "I am one of the only ones doing that docket, so there weren't very many people to choose from."

As hard as you work to get to the level you have achieved, I bet you, like Jessica here, don't take compliments well. You downplay or minimize your greatness. You probably rock your industry often with your awesomeness, but you just can't see it or are just uncomfortable with attention being placed on you.

While you don't acknowledge your accomplishments, you might make your mistakes a bigger deal than they really are, also taking away from the good that might have occurred despite it or even because of it. Either way, your own distorted thinking can contribute to anxiety, low self-esteem, and mood disturbance.

POINTS TO PONDER:

Find someone who knows you well and ask them to tell you three things that they like about you. You are not allowed to respond until they are done. Pay attention to your thoughts during this activity. Write down what you think about and feel in that moment versus what they say about you.

NOTES

NOTES

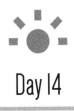

Day 14

MAKING "ALWAYS" AND "NEVER" REGULAR PARTS OF CONVERSATION

Kevin and his wife are having some relationship stress over her lack of support for his playing bass in a band on weekends and evenings. One night, she did not attend what he described as "a very important gig" because she had to work. An argument ensued and he yelled, "You have never supported me in this" and stormed out of the house.

How many times have you, like Kevin, fallen into the trap of using the words "always" and "never" when talking about something negative that is happening with you. The truth is, there are very few things that either *always* happen or *never* happen, yet we use these terms frequently. You take isolated incidents and make them the norm instead of seeing them for what they are.

This dysfunctional thinking distorts your reality and leads you to believe that you are destined for doom. Not only will it detach you from others because you always blame them, but it will also prevent you from taking chances in your life and career. You might not apply for that promotion or not volunteer for a certain committee because you convince yourself that you will "never" get that position because you "always" get looked over anyway or you are somehow unworthy.

POINTS TO PONDER:

Pay attention to your conversation for the next twenty-four hours and try to identify when you or others use the words "always" or "never." Is it the appropriate use of the word? If not, identify an alternative way of stating that sentence.

NOTES

NOTES

Tackling Dysfunctional Thoughts Continued

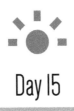

Day 15

MIND READING AND FORTUNE TELLING

John is a third-year medical student on his psychiatry rotation. When preparing for rounds, he states to his peers, "Dr. Jones thinks I'm an idiot. I can tell by the way she looks at me." There is no evidence to support this and Dr. Jones is typically cordial to all of the students. Still, John is anxious about rounds and fumbles when the doctor arrives, having a hard time staying organized.

John became a mind reader. He made the assumption that the attending physician thought he was an idiot despite there being no evidence to support this. Then, he acted agitatedly because of it. This is a prime example of thoughts having a direct effect on behavior and negatively affecting functioning. Making assumptions about what others think is a dangerous path to travel. You could absolutely be correct, but you could absolutely be wrong.

These are times when, as professionals, you need to rely on your team, people who you run these thoughts by in confidence and will give you honest opinion about the situation. In this case, John could have asked the other students if they thought Dr. Jones treated him any differently instead of just stating that she thought he was an idiot. Another tactic would be to pay attention to the situation and make note of evidence to either support or refute your thoughts. You'd be pleasantly surprised by how wrong you are.

POINTS TO PONDER:

Think of someone in your personal or professional life you think doesn't like you or has negative thoughts about you. List specific examples that

support your claim and specific examples that refute your claim. Does the evidence support you? Is
it possible that you are wrong?

NOTES

NOTES

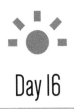

Day 16

NAME CALLING

Sophia is a weekend news anchor who has been asked to fill in for the regular news anchor and is told that there will be a local pet shelter coming in to bring animals who need to be adopted. She immediately tells the co-anchor, "I'm such a loser. I hope I don't mess this up."

Oftentimes, these names we call ourselves roll off our tongue without us even thinking about it or being aware of it because we do it so frequently. Sophia has referred to herself as a loser and I'd bet this isn't the first time. How often have you called yourself names like loser, dork, or idiot after making a mistake? How can you possibly be successful when those are the words that you consistently use to describe yourself? How can you focus and give 100% when you have already defeated your own self with the name calling?

You may be a little clumsy at times but you are not a loser, dork, or idiot. These identities can also be placed onto other people when we call them names. They cloud our view of them and unfairly define them as the names we call them, instead of us actually conceptualizing them as people who sometimes make mistakes (again, everyone does) and/or do things that we don't like.

POINTS TO PONDER:

→ What types of names are you guilty of using on yourself? If you can't think of any, ask those around you. They may be able to identify names you use without even noticing. Write down the words you call yourself and then define them. Don't forget to write those definitions down. Are they accurate descriptions of who you are? Are they accurate descriptions of the people you are describing?

NOTES

NOTES

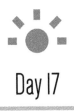

Day 17

THINKING TOO HIGHLY OF YOURSELF

Jacob is one of the new partners in the practice. The holidays are approaching and he is scheduled to work Thanksgiving, which was established several months ago. But at the last minute, he cancels and states that he doesn't think he should have to work the holiday because, based upon the most recent finance report, he had the highest revenue over the past few months. Aside from that, Jacob has also been constantly heard talking about his possessions and comparing them to those of other physicians in the practice.

When you are really good at something or have achieved a high level of status in a given industry, it can get your head. While confidence is great, there is a fine line between confidence and arrogance. Sometimes, the most successful professionals walk very closely to that line, which can get them into trouble. An inflated sense of self may make you think that you've achieved all there is to achieve so you become complacent. You may also stop responding to feedback because you think you don't need it.

Unfortunately, people who think too highly of themselves lack not only insight into themselves, but also lack people to tell them when they are crossing the line from confidence to arrogance. This can easily lead to disastrous interpersonal conflicts in the workplace.

POINTS TO PONDER:

◉ It's time to check yourself! Do you have people in your life who love you enough to tell you when you are getting a little too sure of yourself?

⊙ Do you find yourself looking down on co-workers and being critical of their work?

⊙ Do you find yourself comparing your productivity, products, or sales to your peers and making jokes about your superiority?

NOTES

NOTES

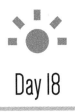

Day 18

INFLEXIBILITY TO OTHER POINTS OF VIEW

Janine and Sarah, both physicians on the medical staff of a small clinic, are responsible for choosing what the medical staff will do this year for their holiday community service event. They cannot agree on which community agency to support and the debate becomes heated. Janine would like to support a local agency that provides confidential medical care to young girls. Sarah, a devout Catholic, refuses to support this agency due to the fact that they provide birth control to girls and this goes against her religious beliefs. As a result of the conflict, the two stop speaking to each other and the clinic staff goes to the medical director with reports of how hostile the work environment has been.

Yikes! This is sticky. While most will agree that it is probably best to avoid politics and religion in the workplace, sometimes, these things come up and you can't avoid it. There is no doubt that certain topics evoke intense emotions and can lead you to react in a less-than-professional way, such as extreme stubbornness about your point of view and irritability. You may also alienate a peer or group of peers and create a hostile work environment.

You are human. Emotions and conflicts happen. You may not be able to control the emotions that you feel, but you definitely have control over how you react to the conflict.

Having the ability to look at conflict from the other point of view is a valuable, beneficial skill that allows you to gain insight into the other person's value and belief system while giving you the opportunity to become acutely aware of your own. Respecting a person's point of view, without necessarily adopting it, can also help with conflict resolution and negotiation, not to mention team-building when you reach consensus or peaceful conclusions Who knows? You may even change your initial way of thinking if you just listen.

Here are some tips to help you gain insight into another person's point of view:

- ⊙ Once conflict arises, pause. If you have to step away and return to the conversation later, please do so. Acting quickly and emotionally can be problematic.

- ⊙ Listen to not only the words that are being used but the emotion that the other person is experiencing.

- ⊙ Restate what you have heard calmly to make sure that you have a firm understanding of what the other person is saying.

- ⊙ When appropriate, provide some of your own thoughts on the conversation. Don't be afraid to share any experiences that may be relevant to the topic.

➲ Thank the person for being willing to have such a difficult conversation with you.

➲ End the conversation completely and clearly. One of you may have a change of opinion or you may agree to disagree. You have at least learned another point of view and gained some insight into what is important to that person.

POINTS TO PONDER

➲ When was the last time you held a conversation with someone who held a different belief system than you?

➲ When was the last time you had a debate about a hot-button topic that left you angry?

➲ Did you listen to each other or were you too busy trying to get your points across?

NOTES

NOTES

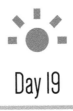

Day 19

ASSUMPTIONS THAT EVERYONE IS LIKE YOU

Janice is an attorney, who happens to be working with a new paralegal today for the first time. She sees that the new paralegal is married and asks what her husband does for a living. The paralegal responds that she is indeed married but that she has a wife, not a husband. This leads to awkward silence and a palpable tension for the rest of the day. The paralegal asks to be reassigned out of concern that she may not be well received by Janice, who made unsettling previous comments about homosexuals prior to learning about the paralegal's sexual orientation.

You know what they say about assumptions! It should never be assumed that the person you are interacting with falls into any particular demographic category or has the same thoughts on topics as you do. This applies to patients, clients, and coworkers. The temptation is to assume that everyone is like us, especially if we find ourselves in the majority category. We may also expect that others will share our viewpoint on issues.

I live in Oklahoma. It would be shortsighted of me to assume that every new patient I see is heterosexual and Christian because most of the state is heterosexual and Christian. It would also be wrong of me to assume that people share similar political or religious views as I do just because we have other things in common. These views affect how we see the world and affect our viewpoint on most issues.

Making assumptions can lead to awkward outcomes and possibly offend the other party depending upon the situation. This could also lead to frustrations on your part and increases in stress when interacting with others. And let's face it, relationships are everything. Remember that this has nothing to do with your stance on their thoughts, but more so about grasping the concept of them having the right to live whatever life they choose and to be respected without it creating conflict. Despite my best efforts, sometimes, I still make the mistake and verbalize an incorrect assumption about someone. When that happens, I immediately apologize for the mistake and move on as best as I can without putting my foot in my mouth yet again.

Here are some communication tips to avoid making assumptions:

- ⊙ Avoid questions that put people into a particular demographic category such as "What does your husband do?"

- ⊙ Speak in more open-ended ways such as "Tell me about your significant other," allowing the other person to provide what details they choose to provide.

➲ If you happen to slip and ask a question that could be offensive, don't hesitate to apologize for the assumption. Simply say, "I apologize for that. How shortsighted of me to assume that."

➲ Avoid stating opinions that could be deemed controversial in the workplace, especially on highly charged topics surrounding politics and religion.

POINTS TO PONDER:

➲ Has anyone ever made an assumption about you based upon some external characteristic that wasn't true? If so, what emotions did that evoke?

➲ Do you often share opinions with others on potentially controversial topics such religion, sexual orientation, or politics without knowing their stances? What problems could this lead to?

NOTES

NOTES

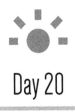

Day 20

REFUSING TO ADMIT YOU ARE WRONG

Nicholas is a pediatrics resident who was supposed to write an order for a patient to have a different pain medication. He became busy and it slipped his mind. While rounding with the attending physician, it came up that the medication hadn't been changed. When asked what happened, he told a drawn out lie that ultimately put the blame on someone else.

The inability to admit to a mistake or to being wrong is complicated. It can come from a simple place of just not wanting to deal with the backlash of your mistake or it could also be affected by what admitting a wrong can mean to an individual. For some, it can be interpreted as admitting to incompetence. While we know that everyone makes mistakes and that one mistake does not equal incompetence, we many not apply that same logic to ourselves in such situations.

A consequence of telling the truth may very well be punishment of some sort, but there are also potential positive benefits to being honest. First and foremost, you can avoid a lot of guilt and sadness that comes from lying or smearing the blame on someone else. Second, you could gain a level of respect with peers and superiors and come across as someone who can be trusted. Most high-level professionals are leaders at some level and being able to admit a wrong can allow you to gain a bit of equity with those you lead.

When admitting to a mistake, be clear and concise about what exactly you are apologizing for; generic apologies are rarely seen as sincere. Then, explain how you will make things right and how you plan to avoid similar mistakes in the future.

POINTS TO PONDER

- Do you have difficulty admitting that you are wrong?

- What are you afraid will happen if you do admit that you were wrong or made a mistake?

NOTES

NOTES

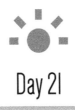

Day 21

THE PROBLEM *MUST* BE EVERYONE ELSE

Johnathan, a surgeon, describes himself as a loner. Ever since college, he has had difficulty forging meaningful relationships. This was evident in medical school, residency, and now as an attending physician. He is typically abrasive with peers, can hardly get along with nursing staff, and usually has conflict with administrators. This is his third attending position since completing residency four years ago and he doesn't appear to be happy. He constantly complains about the level of incompetence of everyone around him and has mentioned of starting a new job search.

Sometimes, you are the problem! You are the reason that you can't get along with anyone! This possibility should be high on your list if you have the same problems interacting with different people across different settings. Not being able to recognize your role can create a toxic work environment for all involved, leading to irritability and anxiety for those affected, as well lack of career fulfillment and depression for the individual.

Here are some signs that you are the common denominator in your workplace unhappiness:

- You find people you work with to be incompetent, especially your superiors.

- You are having difficulty engaging with peers at work.

- You think that you are being lied to or mistreated.

- You have had similar problems with previous employers.

POINTS TO PONDER:

- ❯ Do you tend to have conflict in the workplace with multiple people?

- ❯ Do those who report to you often complain about you?

- ❯ Have you had formal complaints filed about you in the workplace?

- ❯ Is it possible that you contribute to this environment? Is so, what can you do to fix it?

NOTES

NOTES

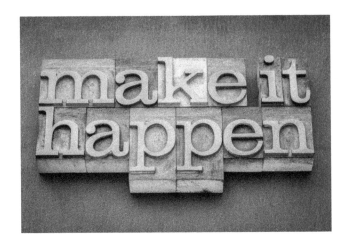

Time for Action

You've learned about basic psychiatric disorders and concepts, and you've spent time identifying a variety of dysfunctional thoughts that can have negative effects on your overall mental health and functioning in the workplace. Now, it's time to develop solutions to combat the problems that you identified in weeks 2 and 3.

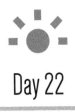

Day 22

SELF-CARE FOR THE BUSY PROFESSIONAL

What do you think of when you hear the term "self-care?" I tend to think of self-care as the art of attending to the distinct needs of the entire self (mentally, spiritually, physically, and relationally) in an effort to achieve a maximum level of overall health. This doesn't mean that you must engage in activities focused on yourself at all times. What it does mean is that you are aware enough of yourself and your needs that you are able to identify which part of yourself needs to be attended to and when. That is the art of the process!

For most high-level professionals, financial constraints do not stop them from engaging in self-care. For most, it will be the time or lack thereof. It can feel overwhelming to fit time in to engage in self-care when you are already so busy with work, family, and other obligations. For others, it may be stigma. You may be acutely aware that you are dealing with an issue for which you should be seeking professional help, but you are too embarrassed to do so because of the way mental health issues are viewed in our society. Guilt or shame may be yet another reason for not seeking out opportunities to engage in self-care: you may be so caught up with work that time for family or friends is limited and it can feel very selfish to engage in self-care activities.

When these reasons get in the way, it's helpful to look at the reasons why you should engage in self-care activities. Taking care of yourself can be one of the best things you can do for not only yourself, but also the people you care about. When you aren't in a good space or you neglect yourself, you can be more irritable and less desirable to be around. This can have negative effects on your most important relationships.

Engaging in self-care is also critical for your health. It can improve sleep patterns, which will, in turn, improve your functioning and overall physical health, decreasing the onset of disorders such as hypertension and diabetes or decreasing the burden of those disorders if you already have them.

Lastly, self-care activities just make you feel good and helps you to clear out some of the negative stuff that can cloud your thoughts. Below is a list of self-care ideas that you can use to get started. By no means is this an exhaustive list. Just a place to get you started if you can't figure out what to do:

- ● Exercise: Being physically active for just thirty minutes a day can help improve sleep, give you more energy to be effective, and improve overall health. If you don't always have thirty minutes to give, do it as many days per week as you can, paying attention to those times when you need it more.

➲ Laugh a little: Allow yourself to have fun! Sometimes those of us who have accomplished a lot have a difficult time relaxing. Laughter truly is good for the soul. It can help improve your mood and relieve stress. So watch a comedy, take a few minutes to watch a funny video online, or let your kids tell you a joke!

➲ Take up a hobby: Find something that you have always wanted to do. Learning new skills is healthy for your brain and it can be very satisfying to master a new skill.

➲ Outsource some things: Sometimes, busy professionals are guilty of doing too much. If there is something that you can realistically do to take some things off your plate, do it. If it is financially feasible and would benefit you to pay a housekeeper to come in just once a month to free you for a day of self-care, it would be well worth it for you and your loved ones. If you can subscribe to a meal-planning service one week out of the month or if you can create a carpooling schedule with other parents, you will gain some valuable time for yourself.

- ⊙ Go outside during the work day: I know this sounds like a minute thing, but you would be surprised by how much better you'll feel after five minutes of sunlight. After all, sunlight can increase serotonin levels.

- ⊙ Take lunch: This means actually take a lunch. Don't eat at your desk. It can be beneficial to step away from work, go eat, and come back refreshed. Even if you just bring your lunch and go outside on a nice day away from your desk, you will see the benefits.

- ⊙ Intentional relaxation: This can be prayer, meditation, mindfulness exercises, or anything that causes you to relax. It must be intentionally planned or else you will be in danger of not doing it as often as you would like to.

➲ Deal with your thoughts and emotions: Sometimes, the best thing you can do for yourself is to step back, take some time to recognize what your emotions and thoughts are doing, and work on you.

NOTES

NOTES

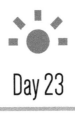

Day 23

GIVE YOURSELF PERMISSION TO BE BROKEN

This one is tough. Most of you have gotten to where you are in life because you worked very hard to get there and you fought through a lot. You have overlooked your own needs and wants to reach a certain level and now you are here. But some of you are broken!

Overachievers tend to function at high levels so it may be difficult for others to notice when you are off of your game, unless you have a severe impairment. But, oftentimes, you yourself know when you aren't well. You may not be as productive as you'd like to be. You may find yourself having less control of your emotions than you typically do. You may even find yourself going through the motions of life and not feeling as if you are really in it. This is when you have to give yourself permission to be broken so that you can work on the repair process.

Don't be so hard on yourself about it either. It is very hard for high-achieving people to accept difficulties like this because, for most of you and your careers, this isn't viewed as acceptable. I can assure you that you are not the first person to need some help putting things back together and you won't be the last. You may be beating yourself up because you see this as a sign of weakness. In reality, it truly does take more courage and strength to say that you are not well and that something needs to be done about it than to suffer in silence.

Allow yourself to not have total control over all situations. There are parts that you can control, but some parts are outside of your control and those are what you struggle with. When you put a lot of energy and effort into changing something that you don't control, you will typically fail. That feeling of failure will lead to you feeling defeated and have a negative effect on your mood and your self-esteem. Give yourself permission to focus on the things that you can actually change and to let those other things go—accept that you can't do it all!

I promise that letting go can be a very rewarding process. If you can identify the problem, take action, and see results, you will feel good about yourself. Most of your careers and minds are result-oriented, so this will put you right in your wheelhouse. Take the time to celebrate this process and all that you accomplish every day!

NOTES

NOTES

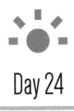

Day 24

DAILY GRATITUDE AFFIRMATIONS

One of the best things that you can do to combat negative thoughts and attitudes is to incorporate gratitude affirmations into your day. Gratitude affirmations are simply statements that you make about things that you are grateful for. Don't overthink this at all. Your gratitude affirmations are yours and can be as big or as small as you want them to be. These affirmations will serve as reminders of the things that make you fortunate. It is easy to get bogged down in the messes of life, so these statements allow you to maintain a sense of clarity and perspective.

Not only can gratitude affirmations give you a sense of perspective, but they can also help in other ways, for you and for others. Actively engaging in gratitude affirmations daily can help improve your stress level. It's difficult to stress about unimportant things when you are actively reminding yourself of the things you are grateful for. Since you will also be highlighting your positives during your gratitude affirmations, you will see more focus and motivation, which can lead to more productivity. When you shift your mindset and challenge what you've always thought about yourself and your life, you will achieve a level of individual growth.

Your attitude of gratitude can also leave a huge mark on the people who come in contact with you on a regular basis. Gratitude can be infectious and you will attract those who are also grateful. Being more grateful will also cause you to be a kinder person and that can only help with established relationships. Nothing's better than to be close to someone who is grateful for your friendship.

Make a plan to be intentional about your gratitude affirmations. It doesn't have to be complicated, but if you want some detailed gratitude exercises, there are tons out there. I tend to stay simple with my gratitude affirmations because it can be hard to find time to do a more involved project—I would probably never do it and would miss out on the benefits of it.

Here are a few simple gratitude affirmation activities that you can do. Do them as frequently as you like!

- ➲ Create a gratitude wall in your office. Write affirmations of gratitude on sticky notes and put them somewhere in your workspace. I keep mine on the inside of a cabinet that nobody sees but me. At least a few times a week, I write something about my job that I am grateful for and, when I am having a bad day at work, I go to that wall. You can do the same thing with your significant other, friends, or children.

⊙ Find time to tell your kids and significant others something about them that you appreciate. I recommend this at least once a week.

⊙ Create a gratitude calendar. Plan out a calendar and assign a different person to each week. Contact that person at least once during that week to tell them something about them that you are thankful for. This is especially handy for those relationships that we value but aren't able to put in as much time as we'd like to.

⊙ While brushing your teeth at night, take a little time to highlight something in your day that was positive and express gratefulness for the opportunity. This can feel a little weird at first but it will be a great exercise.

NOTES

NOTES

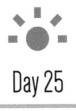

Day 25

BOUNDARY SETTING

Robert Frost said it best in the "Mending Wall": "Good fences make good neighbors."

Boundaries are barriers or lines that we draw to protect ourselves from being treated in ways that we don't desire. In psychiatry, we tend to think of boundaries in terms of borders between people. Setting boundaries comes with identifying what it is that you will accept and won't accept. It should also include setting consequences as to what will happen if those are violated. While these lines do separate us in certain ways, they also have the ability to bring us closer together. It is very important for high-level professionals to have boundaries in personal relationships, but I am going to focus on work relationships in this chapter.

You spend a lot of time at work and the people you work with; in fact, you may spend more time with coworkers than you do with your own family! Boundaries are immensely important in the work place, especially for those in leadership positions. You have the ability to set the tone and expectation for your setting, not to mention the responsibilities that come with being in a position of power that can pressure others without you even trying. The types of boundaries you set will trickle down to those that work below you.

When establishing boundaries, it is important to be firm and assertive without being rude. If you have a coworker who likes to yell at meetings or constantly interrupts you during conversations, you can deal with this without being rude, especially if that just isn't who you are. Simply state, "If you continue to yell at me, I will not have this conversation with you. If this continues, I will report it to someone." In this scenario, you must be willing to carry through on your stated consequence and you must be willing to report it if the boundary-crossing continues. If you have no actual plans of sticking to the boundaries set, you are probably better off not setting them until you are ready to take action. Although some obvious things like yelling are obviously unacceptable, your boundaries should always be clear in every situation and not be open to interpretation by the receiving party. If it is in your best interest to say no to something or someone, do so clearly and concisely. If you hem and haw, the other person may become confused or upset because they misunderstand you. Learning to say no is a great skill!

Setting boundaries fails when you are unclear, too complex in the boundary, or find yourself being too loose or too inflexible. When you aren't clear and resolute in your boundary setting, it appears that you aren't sure of yourself or that you don't know what you need or want. If they are too loose, they rarely provide any protection to either party and are not beneficial at all. Reversely, if you present a boundary that is too complicated, the other person may not be able to follow all of the caveats of the boundary or you yourself may not be able to keep up with own your rules. Some boundaries such as those that involve physical violence should be inflexible and rigid and non-negotiable, but most things do not fall in this category: be mindful of that when setting extremely inflexible boundaries.

Also think about setting boundaries with your career. People who have achieved success professionally have a tough time separating themselves from that identity. But you are not your career and your career doesn't define you. You may have poor boundaries with your career if:

- You rely heavily on your performance at work to achieve happiness.

- You are unable to step away from work long enough to enjoy your family and friends. Can you stop yourself from checking work emails or taking non-urgent calls at dinner?

⊙ You have difficulty finding a sense of fulfillment and wholeness outside of work

Being able to establish healthy boundaries with
work can not only nurture relationships outside of
work, but can also help you define who you are and
what your true needs are as a person.

NOTES

NOTES

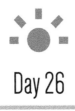

Day 26

DEVELOPING YOUR SUPPORT TEAM

People need people, and you are no different. Even you who has achieved a lot in life. Especially you! With that being said, you must be strategic about who is included in your support team. Your team will consist of family, close friends, and colleagues. You must define what it is that you require of each of them or what value they bring to you so that you know which group of people you can call on at what time. Without having these parameters defined in your mind, you will find yourself frustrated when you go to the wrong group with the wrong need.

Your family is your family. They love you no matter what and will put up with all of your drive and ambition, even when it interferes with your relationship with them. Of course, this includes your significant other and kids. You will likely have a bit more obligation to them, but what about other family? What about your parents, grandparents, siblings, and others? How well are you keeping up with them and nurturing those relationships? These are the relationships that tend to fall by the wayside, even though these family members tend to love you unconditionally. They also keep you humble and remind you of who you really are and where you came from. If, for some reason, your relationships with your family members are failing, I urge you to consider an immediate intervention. In the end, those are the most precious relationships of all.

Your close friends are just that: friends. They may be people you've known since well before you had a career, maybe even as far back as grade school. They may be people you've connected with in adulthood through church, your significant other, or your children, and you may get together on the weekends or take vacations together. These are personal relationships that reach you on a very real, personal level.

As a busy professional, it is often hard to keep up with these relationships because of how full your plate is. It is possible that distance and time may have separated you from your friends a bit, so you don't talk as often as you used to. Despite the difficulty, these relationships are also valuable. They give you a break from the hustle and bustle of your career and allow you to be you. You may be Dr. X when you are at work, but to them, you are just your regular old self. There is something very comforting in that.

The other people on your team are your colleagues. This will not include every colleague you have ever worked with; in fact, it may not include anyone you have worked with in the past. It could be a colleague you went to medical school or law school with. It could be someone you met at a professional conference and connected with. It could be just one person or a group of people. These people understand your professional struggles and stress in a way that your family and friends will not, and you can often say things to them that you can't say to those you are closest to. Sometimes, you will see things in them that you didn't realize were in yourself until you start talking to them. It is extremely helpful to have someone who lives in your world and understands the unique stresses that come with it.

Knowing when to access each part of your team is going to be invaluable. Think about what your needs are to determine which team member is capable of providing support in that moment. In addition, be conscious of your team members' different backgrounds. If you are a highly-paid professional who comes from a lower socioeconomic status, remain sensitive to your family and friends. They may have difficulty hearing you talk about the stress of building your dream house when they would be thrilled just to build a dream house. Don't talk to your family about how stressed you feel about work when they want to spend time with you *away* from work. Choose conversations for the right people. Regardless of who is on your team, they are valuable!

NOTES

NOTES

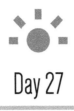

Day 27

CHOOSING YOUR TREATMENT

At this point, some of you have decided that it is time to seek out professional help. Congratulations! Now, let's decide in what setting and at what level.

As mentioned before, general options for treatment settings include inpatient and outpatient. Inpatient treatment of mental health disorders is typically for those with a more severe course of illness who suffer functional impairment. This might include individuals who have suicidal thoughts, especially with plans or intent, or who are unable to care for themselves due to their level of impairment. Inpatient treatment might also be used in the face of extreme tolerability issues with a medication regimen, which requires the aggressive overhaul of a plan.

Outpatient treatment is typically in an office with either a psychiatrist, therapist, or both. Psychiatrists manage medication and can perform psychotherapy in some instances. Therapists are available for psychotherapy. Oftentimes, the recommendation will be to engage in both services. When looking for a board-certified psychiatrist, check factors such as whether or not they take your insurance, if they offer appointments outside of regular hours to accommodate your busy schedule, and what services they offer in office if you prefer to have one provide for both therapy and medication management. When looking into psychotherapy services, be sure to inquire about the types of therapy offered in that practice.

Intensive outpatient services may also be available in your area. These services treat those who require a little more support than what is typically offered in traditional outpatient settings. Participants usually engage in at least a few hours of group therapy for several days per week. This typically occurs for a defined amount of time before transitioning to a traditional outpatient treatment.

Some of you may be on the fence about therapy because you might not feel that you meet a certain level of impairment. There is no baseline level of functioning that you must hit before going to therapy. If you have issues you want to work on, just go! Remember, therapy doesn't have to be a lifetime commitment of weekly sessions on a couch. Therapy can be a couple of months of weekly sessions to help you through a rough patch in your professional or personal life. Anyone who might be having a hard time balancing work and life with subsequent distress can benefit from mental, emotional, and psychological care.

Some of you may be considering treatment for substance use or abuse. If you are addicted to alcohol or anxiolytics (i.e. diazepam, alprazolam, lorazepam, clonazepam, etc.), you may consider inpatient treatment since the withdrawal for those substances—physical and psychological—can be fatal and require medical monitoring. These centers vary on curriculum and time of treatment but can typically last anywhere between thirty and ninety days; once the detox stage is complete, you may consider transferring to an inpatient rehab setting. The goal should be to help you gain understanding of your addiction with emphasis on identification of relapse triggers and how to cope with them once you are discharged.

Outpatient substance use treatment includes support groups like Alcoholics Anonymous, Narcotics Anonymous, or Celebrate Recovery, as well as intensive programs specifically for substance use disorders. Outpatient treatments are also available through a psychiatrist who may prescribe medication to help with cravings or a therapist who performs psychotherapy. Of course, outpatient substance use treatment can be a combination of these things as well.

NOTES

NOTES

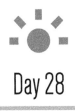

Day 28

CREATING YOUR PLAN

You made it through all 28 days! Now it is time to create your plan for addressing your mental health on an ongoing basis. At this point, you should have a pretty good idea of whether or not you are dealing with a mental illness such as depression or bipolar disorder. If so, seeking treatment should be at the top of your plan's priority list. You should also have a good idea as to which of the negative thought patterns you struggle with the most and hopefully have begun to think of ways to address them.

Now, let's use the topics from Week 4 to complete your plan. The key will be in the scheduling! If it is on your calendar, you are more likely to do it.

SELF-CARE

What are you going to do to address your self-care needs? Your self-care doesn't have to be elaborately planned. It can literally be five minutes of deep breathing in your office between meetings if that is all you can spare. I recommend doing something daily and, if you can't swing daily, do something at least more days of the week than not. I also recommend that you find time in your schedule monthly for at least two extended periods of self-care. That can be having lunch with friends, enjoying spa day, going on a long hike or walk, taking a photography class at the local community college, or whatever it is that you need to recharge. Be sure to physically schedule it in your calendar because, if you don't, it will never happen!

GRATITUDE AFFIRMATIONS

Create a habit of affirming yourself with gratitude every day. Some days it may be about your job. Others may be about acknowledging yourself or something very general. Nothing is too big or small to be grateful for! Just go with it. I recommend that you do this intentionally at first to get into the habit. Try associating the act of affirmation with something that you do daily like brushing your teeth or having your morning coffee. After a while, it will become second nature and you will find yourself doing it all the time. Be grateful for them all.

IDENTIFYING YOUR TEAM

Who is on your team? What steps do you need to take to strengthen those relationships? Pick one person weekly from any of the categories previously discussed (family, close friends, and colleagues) and plan to call them. Choose a time that is typically convenient for you. Maybe Saturday mornings before the kids' activities start or Sunday evenings as you prepare for the week ahead.

NOTES

NOTES

THANK YOU

Thank you so much to my husband and children for always supporting me and believing in me, even when I don't believe in myself. You give me constant motivation to keep pushing and to keep working on myself so that I can be someone who makes you proud. I don't know what I would do without you all. I love you to pieces!

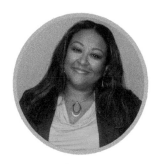

ABOUT THE AUTHOR

Dr. Nicole B. Washington is a board-certified psychiatrist and author. Through her practice, Elocin Psychiatric Services, PLLC, she serves high-level professionals who struggle to accept and treat mental health disorders and other life stressors. She tailors her services to fit the distinct needs and schedules of busy working men and women so that they may enjoy a better quality of life.

Dr. Washington earned her doctor of osteopathic medicine from Oklahoma State University College of Osteopathic Medicine and her master's degree in public health from the University of Illinois,

Chicago. She currently resides in Broken Arrow, Oklahoma, with her husband and two children.

To connect, visit her website at
www.drnicolepsych.com

CREATING DISTINCTIVE BOOKS
WITH INTENTIONAL RESULTS

We're a collaborative group of creative masterminds
with a mission to produce high-quality books to position
you for monumental success in the marketplace.

Our professional team of writers, editors, designers,
and marketing strategists work closely together to ensure
that every detail of your book is a clear representation
of the message in your writing.

Want to know more?
Write to us at info@publishyourgift.com
or call (888) 949-6228

Discover great books, exclusive offers, and more at
www.PublishYourGift.com

Connect with us on social media

@publishyourgift